REIKI

ENERGY

Discover the Ancient Arts of Self-Healing the
Mind and Body

M.E. Dahkid

ISBN-10: 1502537370
ISBN-13: 978- 1502537379

DEDICATION

To those in pursuit of a natural form of healing that allows
the attuned person to heal themselves or others by
channeling the universal life force energy through them
and pass this energy on to self-heal or heal others.

CONTENTS

INTRODUCTION

You use your hand for many things, which can include healing. Hands do not have to be pushing or slapping, but simply gently resting can bring relief and comfort.

The history of medicine shows one of the most difficult things to try to understand is how the human body heals. To date medical science does not have the answer. Professional medical care is not replaceable in any physical or mental crisis, but Reiki complements medical care and helps with the side effects of all medical treatments.

Reiki is a natural form of healing that allows the attuned person to heal themselves or others by channeling the universal life force energy through them and pass this energy on to self-heal or heal others. Reiki can be used to help heal oneself or others in need. It does not require any special talent or magical formula; instead the person who wishes to channel the universal life force energy only needs to be attuned by a Reiki Master or Reiki Master Teacher in order to open up the pathway to healing. It is not religious based and can be practiced by anyone who chooses to be attuned to the energy.

CHAPTER 1 – UNDERSTANDING REIKI ENERGY

Many people are not familiar with the practice and method of Reiki Energy Therapy. Nonetheless, Reiki is worthy of study and application as it can be an effective alternative management and treatment to self-heal the mind and body.

Various diseases and illnesses have invaded mankind since time immemorial. Along with these, diverse methods and treatments have been discovered to treat such medical conditions. One of these methods is the use of Reiki Energy. However, Reiki is not for the sick only. Those who are well could also benefit a lot from this therapy. It is an untapped potential available for all, whether one is well or sick.

Origin Of Reiki Method

Reiki is a combination of two Japanese and Chinese words or characters - Rei and Ki. Rei, which means universal, pertains to that which is unseen or a spirit. Ki is life energy (others call it God, Buddha, Chi, Qi, or Prana). In the early 1920's, a lay monk by the name of Mikao Usui from Japan started of the practice we now know as Reiki. Usui believed that human beings possessed, and at the same time, surrounded with subtle forms of life energy. When these energies are blocked or become lower in amount, the person becomes sick or ill. Reiki Energy would then provide the balance for the human energy fields called as "Auras" and energy centers known as "Chakras".

Usui taught around 2,000 students about his spiritual beliefs on how to heal themselves and others. Through the process termed as "attunements", Usui was able to transfer his healing power to other people as they became masters of Reiki themselves. He had 16 Reiki masters during his lifetime.

One of the original 2,000 students was Chujiro Hayashi, who through the help and guidance of Usui, opened a Reiki clinic in Tokyo. In this clinic, Hawayo Takata sought treatment and was healed of various ailments. Takata became a devoted student of Reiki in the process. It was she who brought the Reiki practice to Hawaii where she was based, and then later on, in the US Mainland. Takata was able to produce 22 Reiki masters. Today, Reiki is widely recognized and accepted worldwide as an alternative treatment to different medical conditions affecting mankind.

Reiki – The Healing Art

Reiki is a healing art that utilizes the technique of the ancient laying-on of hands to heal individuals, whatever their condition might be. It is founded on the belief that life energy force can be transferred from one person to another to balance the energies within the sick person. The healing energies can be released from the practitioner's body through the palms and hands to flow into the recipient's body. These life energies are inexhaustible and have healing powers. These energy fields can be balanced by energy therapies such as touch. Unlike other alternative treatments, Reiki addresses not only the physical health of an individual but also the emotional, mental and spiritual.

People avail of Reiki treatments for different reasons. Some healthy individuals practice or receive Reiki to improve their wellbeing. They are not actually sick but they find Reiki can make them feel even better. Some even find their true purposes in life while undergoing the therapy. Sometimes, major decisions are made after Reiki therapy like moving to a new location, marrying long-time partners, or starting a business. How come? Reiki helps clear the mind and gives a sense of focus and direction. Hopes are also renewed, giving the recipients of Reiki energy new inspirations and aspirations.

People who suffer from chronic pain find relief with the use of this approach, too. People requiring constant medical care because of their chronic illnesses also benefit from the use of Reiki. Cancer patients and those undergoing chemotherapy treatments report a reduction of pain and discomfort.

Reiki is a simple healing practice that can be learned by any individual of any age to benefit oneself or others. The procedure is simple but reports of its effects are enormous. This ancient practice might be the answer that you are looking for today.

M.E. Dahkid

CHAPTER 2 - THE REIKI PRACTICE: AN INTRODUCTION

Reiki is unique as an alternative medicine because of the following features.

1. It is more spiritual than physical. Although this ancient practice is gaining popularity for its ability to relieve people of their medical symptoms, Reiki is more known for its spiritual effects such as inner peace and calm. There is no religious belief system applied to Reiki and yet, those who have practiced and received Reiki claim to have increased sense of connection to their spirituality.

2. It is passive rather than active. Reiki practitioners do not claim that they can diagnose and reorganize the energy fields to heal the individuals. Instead, the practitioners would simply lay their hands on or off the person and the amount of energy released depends on the amount of energy needed by the person. The practitioner has no

power to specify how much energy is to be given to the person. In this way, it is said that Reiki energy is able to customize the necessary amount of energy needed.

3.   It is non-invasive. The therapy does not hurt or do harm to the patient. There is no invasion of privacy in any way. The recipient is fully clothed. This can be done anytime of the day and anywhere. It does not require any tool or machine.

4.   It can be transferred to another person of any age. Through several classes and sessions, Reiki practice can be learned by any individual and applied to another person or to oneself, as the need arises. Actually, Reiki was originally designed as a self-care program. Later on, it has spread as a way to administer help to others who are not well. Today, even healthy individuals take advantage and enjoy the effects of Reiki.

What happens during a Reiki Therapy?

The procedure when one avails of Reiki treatment is very simple. Here is what you can expect to occur when you employ this alternative medicine.

Finding a Reiki master to do the therapy is a very important task. Ask around or check the forums online. You need to have someone whom you can trust. Some hospitals offer this service. You could ask your doctor for any recommendations.

When you are about to start the therapy, the first thing you would notice is the tranquility of the room. This relaxing atmosphere is achieved through dimmed lights, soft music and a soothing aroma. However, there would be some instances where there would be total silence, as some Reiki masters prefer absence of any distractions during therapy.

You would be fully clothed except for footwear. You could do therapy in the clothes that you came in with. However, the preferred attire is loose-fitting garment. Some clinics provide their own hospital gown for patients to wear. The ideal fabrics are natural ones such as wool, cotton or linen. If you are wearing belts or other constricting garments or accessories, the practitioner would request that you loosen or remove them. He or she could also request removal of pieces of jewelry that you have on you. It is best not to wear these at all when you plan to get Reiki therapy.

Depending on the location and practitioner, you would be asked to sign a consent form. There can be instances where you would be asked some questions regarding your current health condition. At this point, you could inform your practitioner of your preferences (whether to lie or sit down, with music or none, if you prefer not to be touched directly, and so on).

You would be asked to lie down. It could be in a bed, a couch or a massage table. For patients with back problems, sitting upright in a chair is allowed. Assume the most comfortable position that you can because you should be completely relaxed. You could either do the breathing exercise technique to soothe your nerves or just close your eyes and empty your mind from worries or anxious thoughts.

The Reiki practitioner would then either touch you directly or just hover their hands two to three inches above your skin. The placement of the hands would be lightly on or above the affected area (fresh wounds would not be touched). The touch is very light and non-intrusive. You should not feel any pressure from the touch. Some practitioners have predetermined sequence on the places where their hands would touch the patients while others follow their "feel" or "leading" where to place their hands. They would let their hands stay on a specific place for two to five minutes. From there, it is expected that the life energy needed would be supplied to the recipient's body. It is then that healing would take place.

There is no protocol when it comes to time of the therapy. Each session could take 15-20 minutes, but there are also times when it would be 90 minutes. Take note however, that this is not a one-time session. Although visible positive effects can occur at any time, Reiki therapy usually takes about four sessions. There is no limit to the number of sessions that you can avail, though. If you want to do this everyday (either on your own or with a practitioner), you could do so.

Some Reiki masters offer home service. If you wish to employ this type of service, arrange your room in such a way that it would be conducive for relaxation. Other than this, the same procedure would apply.

The Reiki Phenomenon

You may have heard of the "phantom hand" phenomenon associated with the Reiki practice. This is the incident where the patient feels that there is another pair of hands touching him or her on a different part of the body. For instance, the practitioner's hands are on the stomach but the patient would feel another pair of hands on the thighs or legs. There are even reports of several hands being felt as if there are many people inside the room although the patient can see the practitioner only.

This phenomenon could be attributed to the concept that the life energy is being transferred and distributed from the Reiki master to the patient. In the process of the transfer and flow of the energy, the sensation is felt. That is why it seems as though there are many hands touching you.

Different sensations

Experience with Reiki therapy is unique for each person. You might hear reports of how "hot" or how "cold" the practitioner's hands were. Do not base your expectations on what you hear from other people. As you go with the therapy, whether it is hot or cold, expect that you would receive what your body needs. In the medical field, both warm and cold could provide healing. It would depend on what is the condition. This is the same with Reiki.

Last Instructions

Other than these, the recipients of these life energies have mostly positive reports about the treatment. Usually, they come out of the treatment revitalized and refreshed. Many claimed that there was indeed healing of the mind and body that took place.

As with all alternative medicines, consultation with your primary provider regarding the use of Reiki practice is recommended. Reiki does not claim to be a substitute for actual medical care. Reiki is designed to complement the outcome of traditional treatment. It aims to assist the individual to gain better health through the self-healing of the body and the mind. If you are undergoing traditional medicine and treatment, continue with these unless instructed by your doctor.

M.E. Dahkid

CHAPTER 3 - MIND-BODY BENEFITS OF REIKI ENERGY

Reiki therapy is a natural healing therapy, which brings health to the people by balancing the energies within them. It has many known benefits. The foremost of which is the reduction of stress and acquisition of inner peace or calmness; for many people, this benefit alone is reason enough to take Reiki therapy.

Stress has been with mankind since day one. Some philosophers have stated that the reason why newborns cry just after being delivered is because they are already stressed. In reality though, stressors (those agents causing the stresses) are neutral. How a person responds to the stress is the main issue. For instance, traffic jams can be taxing to one person but bliss to another. An exam can be frightening to one student but challenging to another. The difference lies on how one perceives the situation or thing – is it a threat or an opportunity?

When the body is stressed, it has its own defense mechanism to protect or preserve itself. There are two probable actions of the body as a system in the face of a stressful event – it would either fight it or run away from it. This is called the fight or flight response. In the process of either fighting or running away from it, the body would either overcome the stress or be exhausted from the process. In Reiki therapy, it assists the individual to overcome stress and achieve a relaxed countenance.

Reiki helps the individual prevail over the harmful effects of stress by creating a peaceful internal environment. When one is at peace within the inner self, then external peace is also achieved. Even though the surrounding is chaotic, the person could remain free from turmoil.

Do you want to know what the absence of or decrease in stress could do to you? Here are some benefits of being free from the hold of stress, which are equivalent to the benefits of Reiki therapy.

1. Healthier heart. Stress is proven to be hazardous to the cardiovascular system of the body. It makes the blood vessels constrict, causing the passage of blood to be lesser than the usual. If such is the case, the vital organs (most especially the heart) and other body parts are greatly affected. Blood pressure tends to go up. The heart's workload is increased. Stress hormones are released, causing the muscles to tense. Since the heart is also a muscle, the harder it works, the bigger it gets, and this can cause a lot of health complications.

    Reiki therapy causes the muscles to relax and the blood vessels to dilate. The results therefore are a healthier heart, lower blood pressure and adequate tissue perfusion (supply of oxygenated blood) to the whole body.

2. Stronger immune system. Your ability to ward off bacteria, viruses and harmful microorganisms is increased when you are relaxed. On the other hand, you tend to have poorer resistance when you are stressed. This is why recipients of Reiki therapy notice that they have fewer incidences of being sick when they practice this healing therapy.

3. Improved sleeping pattern. A relaxed person also gets to enjoy more rest and sleep unlike a tensed person. With more hours of sleep and rest, the body's cells get rejuvenated. Plus, it makes the person less cranky.

4. Lessened pain. Reiki therapy promotes the release of endorphins. These are the hormones of the body that have anesthetic effects. Cancer patients and those with chronic illnesses suffering from pain demonstrate more tolerance to pain as the threshold for pain is increased because of these hormones.

5. The digestive system is also healthier. When a person is stressed, there is increased production of gastric acids, which could irritate and damage the lining of the stomach. Stress also causes difficulty in digesting the food thereby leading to indigestion, stomachaches and upsets. Reiki therapy calms the person leading to a normal process of digestion.

6. Aging process is delayed. One secret of looking young is being stress-free. Wrinkles and facial lines do not form immediately. On the contrary, being less anxious creates a glowing and healthy skin. As there is adequate delivery of blood to all body parts, the integumentary system or the skin (which

is usually the last one to be delivered of oxygenated blood when there is not enough supply) received the needed supply to make it healthy and look good.

These are just some of the physical benefits one could enjoy with Reiki therapy. Reports have been made regarding healing from the following medical conditions: Asthma, migraines, ulcers, arthritis, back problems, minor skin conditions to name just a few.

Emotional and Mental Health

A lot of Reiki patients appreciate the mental rest that the practice provides them. Compared to physical challenges, the mind is oftentimes more challenging to manage. The fatigue that one gets from too much worrying is almost the same as that of a rigorous exercise. With Reiki therapy, there is reduction of mental unrest. Depression can also be prevented.

As the person is less tense, the ability to focus and make sound decisions is enhanced. A clear mind sees all the angles and considers all data before plunging into action or decision. This creates a domino effect with a higher quality of life as the end result.

Additionally, Reiki improves the social aspect of the individual too. As it gives this light feeling within the person, he or he becomes more optimistic. Also, it helps boost the self-confidence. With a positive perspective, relating to other people becomes easier and effortless.

Emotionally and mentally, Reiki also helps the individual achieve peace and calmness. It gives a feeling of joy and hope. It actually makes a person stronger in facing his everyday battles.

There are many benefits of Reiki, indeed. However, are you aware that spiritual healing can occur too because of Reiki? Find out more about this in the next chapter.

M.E. Dahkid

CHAPTER 4- SELF-HEALING OF THE SPIRIT WITH REIKI

Usui, the founder of Reiki therapy was a Buddhist. Nonetheless, in his spiritual teachings about healing, he generalized the presence of a Supreme Being. He did not specify Buddha as the main source of Ki or of the life energy. Takata, on the other hand, has modified the health therapy to include that of the Christians and other beliefs. The Ki could be God, Chi, Qi or Prana.

The concept is simple. There is a Higher Being who possesses the ultimate life force energy. Man has this life force energy but to a certain limit only. When there are blockages to the life force energy within, balance of energies is disrupted. To regain balance, someone who has a deep connection with the Higher Being can transfer some of the needed life force energy coming from the Higher being into the needy individual.

Similar accounts of these healing experiences have been recorded even in the Bible. It has mentioned words as laying-on of hands to the sick too. Plus, the known saints such as Peter and Paul have healed thousands of people through touching the people and transferring the healing power of God into the believers. Jesus Himself laid His hands on the sick and they recovered. Therefore, Reiki therapy is not something new to the Christians. This is why even in the midst of high technology, this ancient healing therapy is still recognized and accepted.

As mentioned, the healthy individuals could also benefit from Reiki. There are also many accounts both in the Bible and other religious books where laying-on of hands is done to transfer the anointing of the master to his follower. This is the reason why Reiki is also being availed by those who are not sick.

Reiki has no attachment to any religion, and yet many of its recipients have received spiritual enlightenment and growth during the process. Why? This phenomenon could be attributed to the fact that there is acknowledgement of a Higher Being, who is the source of the life force energy. This makes the person go back and be more conscious of his relationship with the one that he has faith in.

Part also of the Reiki therapy is cleansing of the mind and freeing it from all negativity and pains. As the person does this, he gets the freedom from past hatred and failures. He realizes his inner hurts. He learns to let go of them and start anew. In the process, one gets to know his inner self deeper. His spirituality is revived.

Healing of the spirit takes place when there is forgiveness and love. When the person lets go of the past, he also let go of the negative experiences. He then turns towards the Higher Being for healing and health. There is purification and cleansing of the inner self. Therefore, inner calm and peace is achieved.

Self-healing of the spirit with Reiki has led many people to rediscover their spiritual passion and real purposes in life. It has strengthened the faith of many recipients. It has removed the fears and doubts in their hearts as they have reconnected in peace with the one whom they consider as divine.

M.E. Dahkid

CHAPTER 5 – BECOMING A REIKI MASTER

When Reiki has touched a person so deeply that he or she is totally attached to it, it would not come as a surprise to have the desire to become a Reiki master. As a Reiki master, one would not only reap benefits for oneself but more importantly, one would be able to help others who need the Reiki energy. The question you may want to know the answer now is how to become a Reiki master? Here are the simple steps.

1. Assess your motivation for this desire. Why would you want to become a Reiki master? Motivation is perhaps the main ingredient to your success as a master. Your reasons could vary. It could be maybe to help and improve yourself more. Or, maybe you want to discover the higher purpose of life.

    Maybe you have a loved one suffering from chronic illness and you want to comfort him through Reiki therapy. It could be that you have experienced what Reiki can do to an individual and you want to share the experience with others, even to strangers. Do not feel condemned that you are also thinking of becoming a Reiki master because you want to set up your own clinic.

Reiki could be a source of income, and there is absolutely nothing wrong with that. It would be wrong though to use Reiki energy to manipulate and abuse other people. Remember, Reiki is also about your faith in the divine. The source of the life force energy is from the Supreme Being and as such, it is all for goodness' sake only.

2.   Assess if you are willing to give time to achieve this desire. Becoming a master could be done in no time at all. There is a course available online and you can finish it according to your own pace. But if you want to be a real special and dedicated Reiki master, you must be ready for several years to "ripen", so to speak. You would be under the guidance of a Reiki master who would initiate and train you to the Reiki way of life. It could sometimes take years.

However, these are not wasted years. These are precious years where you would grow personally and spiritually. Take the time to ripen. Do not think that your desire would wane as the years go by. If you really think that you are called to be a Reiki master, then that desire would continue to burn even with time.

3.   Commit to follow the complete practice of the Usui System. As you go through the process, you would have various opportunities to challenge and questions some of the Usui practices. However, when you truly desire to be a good master, try to

understand the teachings and the ways of the masters. You must be willing to surrender your own will to achieve the full essence of the practice. As a future master, you should abide to the practice and transfer the same practice to other Reiki students later on.

4. Choose carefully the Reiki master who would initiate and guide you. You would be under the guidance of a Reiki master. Select the one whom you trust and can build a lasting relationship with. Choose the one who has mastery of the system, the maturity of a leader, credibility in all areas especially in finances, and someone you have a special connection with. Remember, this initiation and training could take years. Therefore, your master would be like a family member so you have to have someone whom you respect and trust.

5. Attend the classes and internalize the teachings. There are variations of classes being offered. As you search online, you would find different levels, curriculum and lessons. Find out which one is the best for you. Reiki classes have lectures, discussion, demonstrations and actual experiences included in the curriculum.

6. Grow in your knowledge of Reiki. You could do this by building relationships with your classmates and teachers. Associate with other people who could help you understand and learn Reiki therapy. Search for gatherings and meetings and try to attend as many of them as you can. Learning about Reiki does not end after class hours. Continue to meditate and know about it even after class.

7. Apply the teachings to yourself. You do not need to be sick to enjoy the benefits of Reiki energy. As the focus of Reiki is self-healing, be the first one to benefit from your studies. Treat yourself daily; not to heal you of any disease but to increase the depth of self-discovery and spiritual growth. This would also give you the confidence when you start to apply Reiki therapy to other people. As you have first-hand experience with Reiki, sharing and demonstrating to others would be easy.

8. Be ready for opposition. As with all things, there would be controversies and people that you would come across who would discourage you in this endeavor. Be ready for them. Reiki therapy has encountered numerous oppositions from different organizations. Scientists are questioning the veracity of the life force energy.

    Up till today, there is no gadget or machine that could actually measure the energy being released by the master and being received by the patient. Doctors and other medical people could question the healing power of Reiki energy. Sometimes, there would be patients who have received Reiki energy therapy that would comment that it has not done anything for them. These things are expected. However, you do not owe these people any explanation. Reiki therapy works according to one's faith. You cannot possibly hope to please everybody, there would always be opposition. The best thing is to walk in love and demonstrate the real essence of Reiki energy. These energies are meant for good and not to promote strife among people. So focus on the good and not on the bad.

9. Be a student for life. Even when you have

achieved the title of a master, remain teachable and humble. Continue to hone your skills and increase your knowledge on Reiki. Learning is a lifetime process. Understanding the life force energy is not going to happen within a six-month course. Although you would find most online courses to be this short, your personal study should be different.

10. Share to others. Although Reiki initially meant to care for the self, later on, caring for others has become the priority too. Therefore, as you go on with Reiki, share this knowledge to others so that they too, may enjoy its benefits. You would appreciate the inner joy that it would give to you when you see other people benefiting from Reiki energy too. It is priceless to witness a changed life all because you shared this approach to a person.

The desire to become a master of Reiki is a noble desire. Anybody could achieve this when he or she puts her heart and mind to it.

A FINAL WORD

Life with Reiki Energy

Life with Reiki energy is meant to be enjoyed daily. It is not a one-time special occasion where you avail of its benefits and then go back to your previous life as if you have not been touched by it. It is actually life changing. You would not be the same person again. For others, the meaning of life was discovered through Reiki. However, not everybody would be able to say the same. To some people, Reiki therapy would just be another therapy to help them with their current medical condition, nothing more. Where lies the difference? It would fall on how you perceive Reiki.

Reiki is a way of life. Through Reiki, there would be self-discovery and awareness. There would be renewed hope and purpose of life. There would be new promises and inspirations. One would have the aspiration to become better. When you understand the life force energy that is transferred from the practitioner to you, you would know that new life force energy is running your system. You would understand that you are also new now.

With this new revelation, you can look at yourself in a different way. For most people, they get the sensation of feeling unique and special. It is with this revelation that their lifestyle is also changed. They now try to live healthy. They have this desire to abstain from anything that could affect their life energy such as vices, unhealthy habits and wrong company. A higher quality of life is therefore possible now.

Reiki could also change your perspective of what is important and valuable. As it focuses more on the spiritual aspect, the love for material and physical things diminishes. One is more concerned with the inner peace and calm. Life has become simpler, too. Acquisition of material things will not be the main purpose in their lives. Inner peace is.

Reiki makes one more understanding of other people, too. One develops the tolerance to become more patient with others. Dealing with others become easier; you see them as individuals who need the love and care of other people such as yourself. Now that you are filled with love from within, it is easy to give love to others.

Life with Reiki energy is what everybody needs today. You can avail of it. You can enjoy it, today.

Please Leave a Review

Finally, if you enjoyed this book, please take the time to share your thoughts and post a review on Amazon. It'd be greatly appreciated!

That review and feedback will help me improve the content in my books – and make each and every one more relevant and helpful to you.

Thank you again and good luck!

M.E. Dahkid